my mindful day

Yoga

Published in the United States of America by Cherry Lake Publishing
Ann Arbor, Michigan
www.cherrylakepublishing.com

Reading Adviser: Marla Conn, MS, Ed., Literacy specialist, Read-Ability, Inc.
Book Designer: Jennifer Wahi
Illustrator: Jeff Bane

Photo Credits: ©Adamov_d/Shutterstock, 5, 15; ©noprati somchit/Shutterstock, 7; ©EvgeniiAnd/Shutterstock, 9; ©VGstockstudio/Shutterstock, 11; ©pixfly/Shutterstock, 13; ©Hung Chung Chih/Shutterstock, 17; ©Chirtsova Natalia/Shutterstock, 19; ©Aleksey Kurguzov/Shutterstock, 21; ©wavebreakmedia/Shutterstock, 23; Cover, 6, 16, 20, Jeff Bane; Various vector images throughout courtesy of Shutterstock.com

Copyright ©2020 by Cherry Lake Publishing
All rights reserved. No part of this book may be reproduced or utilized in any form or by any means without written permission from the publisher.

Library of Congress Cataloging-in-Publication Data has been filed and is available at catalog.loc.gov

Printed in the United States of America
Corporate Graphics

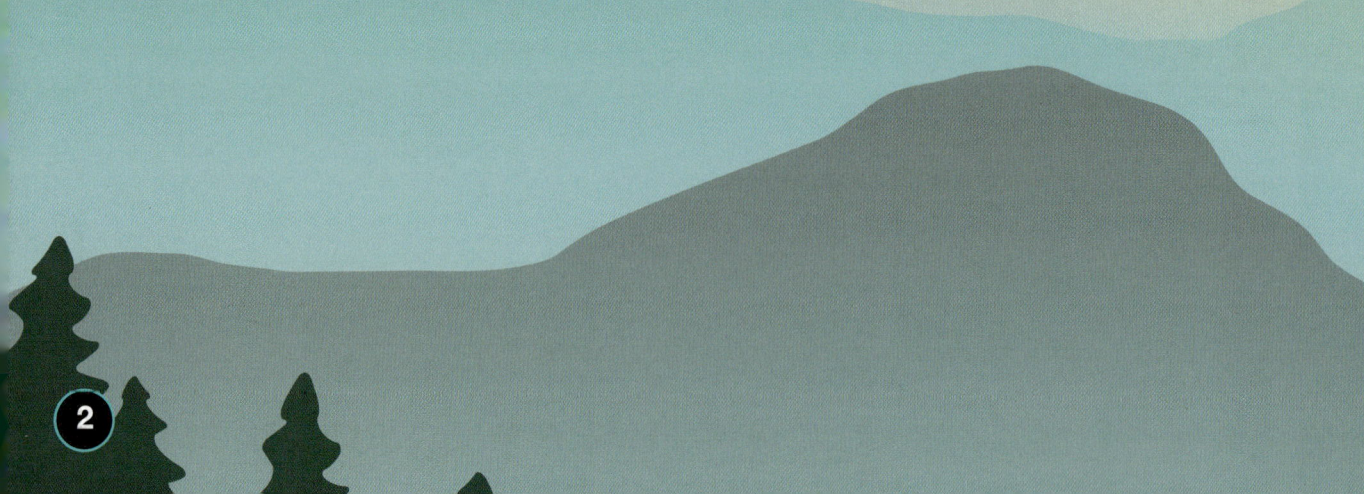

table of contents

Being Mindful 4

Glossary 24

Index 24

About the author: Katie Marsico is the author of more than 200 reference books for children and young adults. She lives with her husband and six children near Chicago, Illinois.

About the illustrator: Jeff Bane and his two business partners own a studio along the American River in Folsom, California, home of the 1849 Gold Rush. When Jeff's not sketching or illustrating for clients, he's either swimming or kayaking in the river to relax.

being mindful

Lay out your mat.

Pick a **pose**.

Breathe in.

Hold it . . .

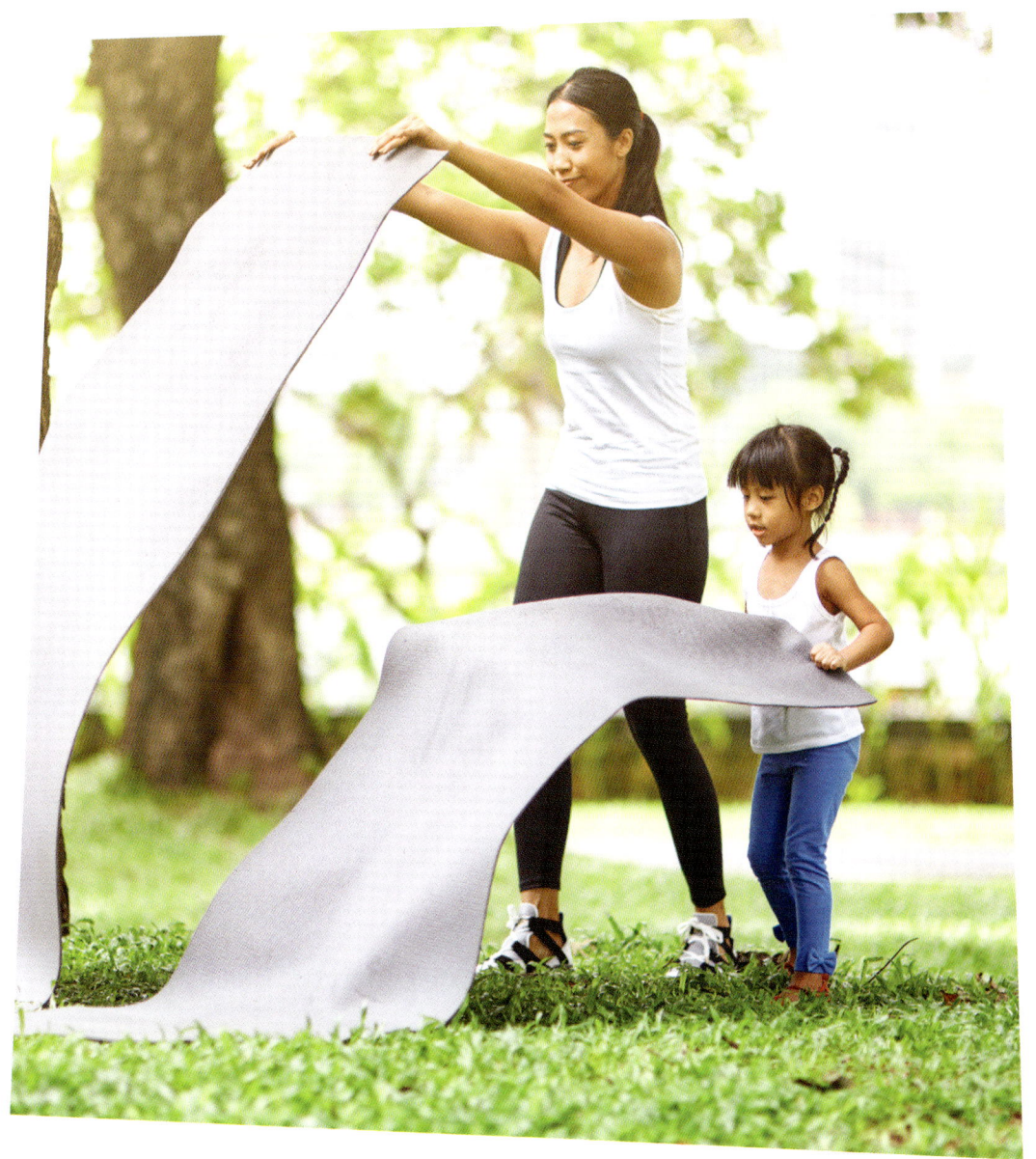

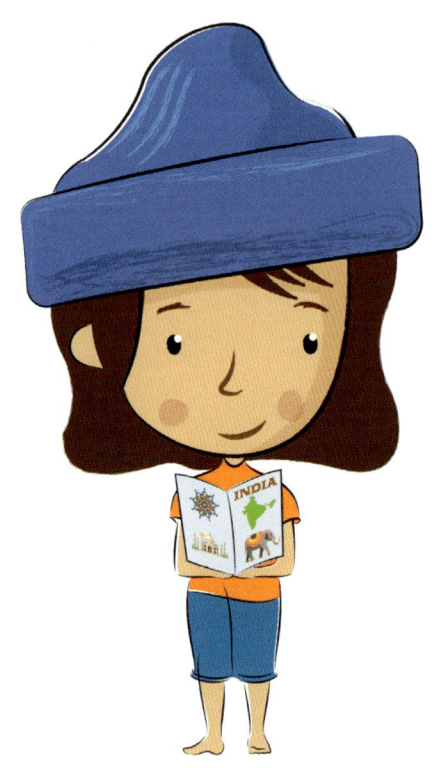

Sound familiar?

Yoga has been around awhile.

It's at least 5,000 years old!

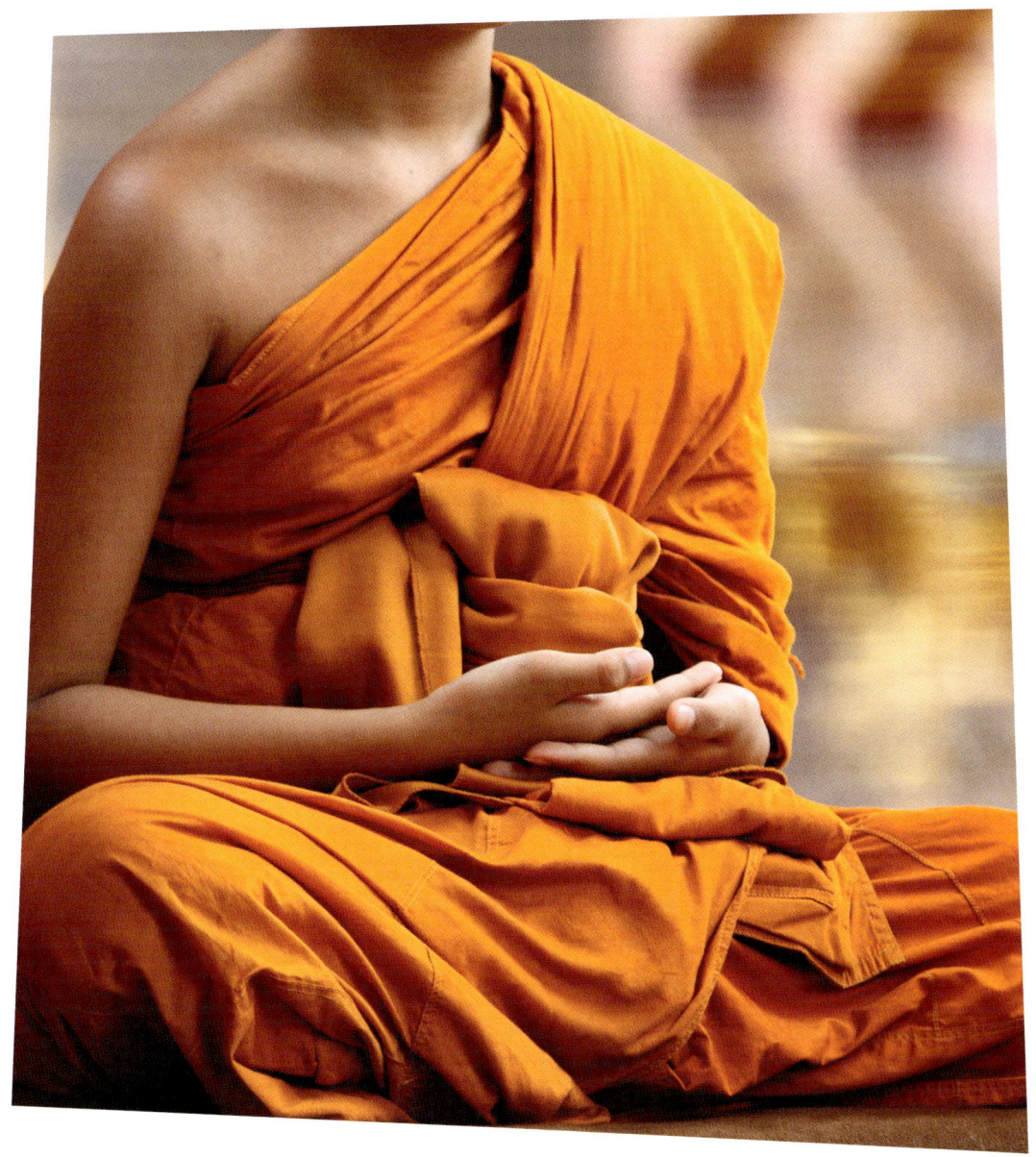

Today, people do yoga to **relax**.

Some see it as exercise.

It's about being happy and having balance.

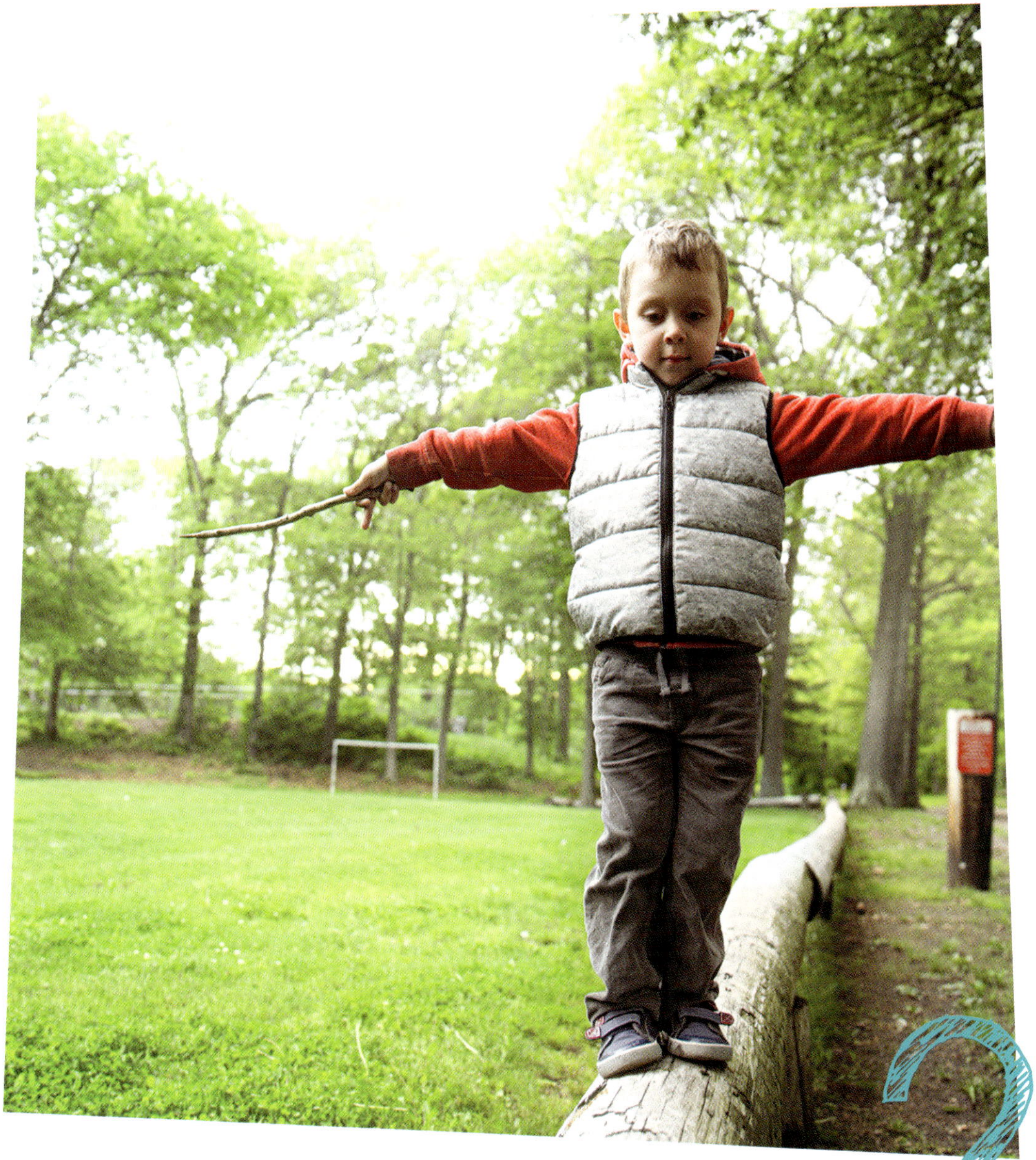

What is your favorite way to exercise?

Yoga keeps your body fit.

It's also good for your mind.

It can help you find **inner peace**.

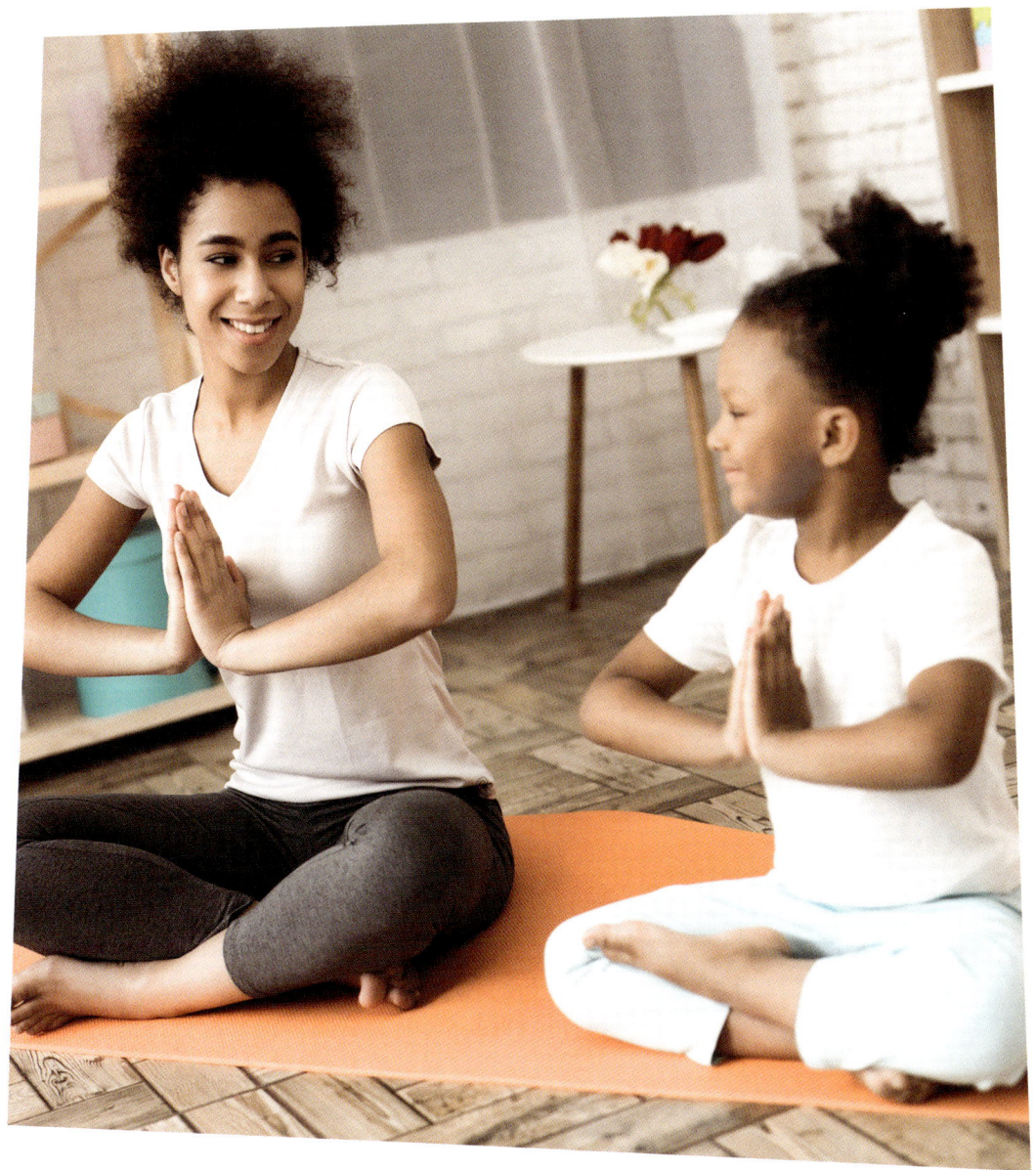

The movements in yoga aren't **random**.

The poses calm you.

They clear your head.

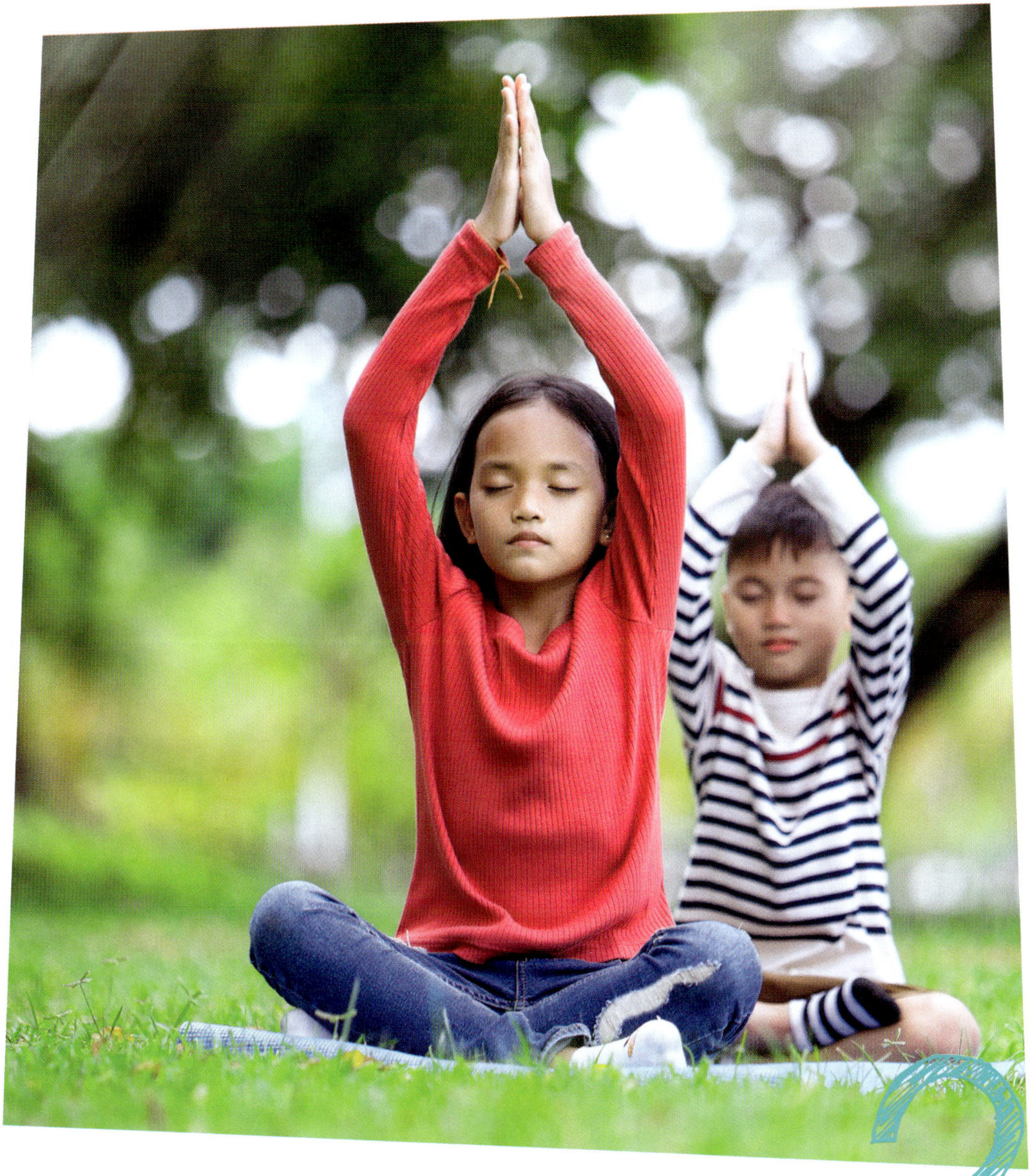

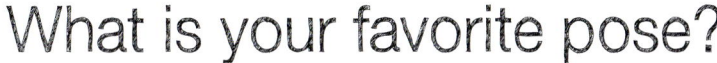
What is your favorite pose?

Yoga helps you **focus**.

It makes you more **mindful**.

Some people **chant** to focus.

Others **meditate**.

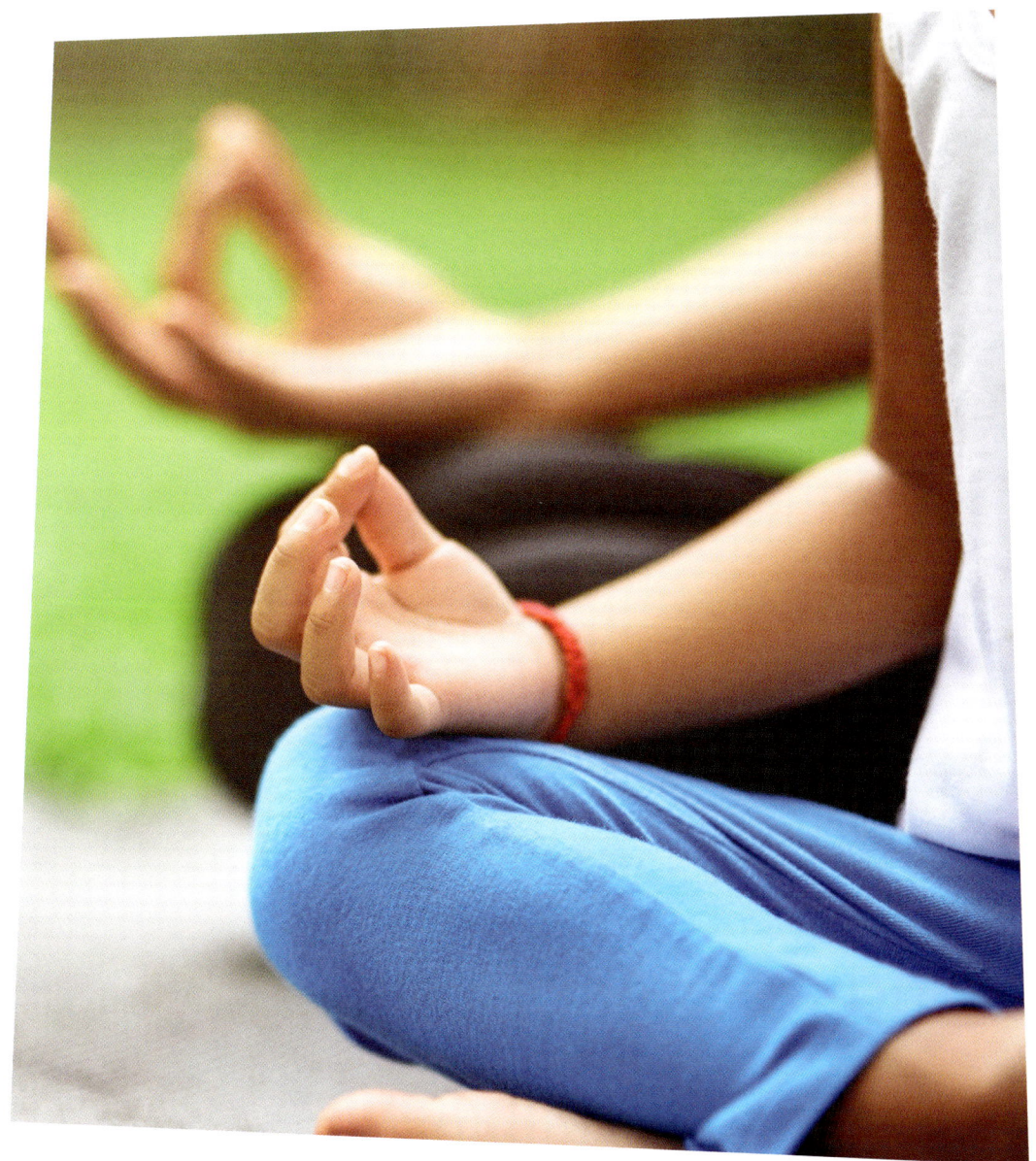

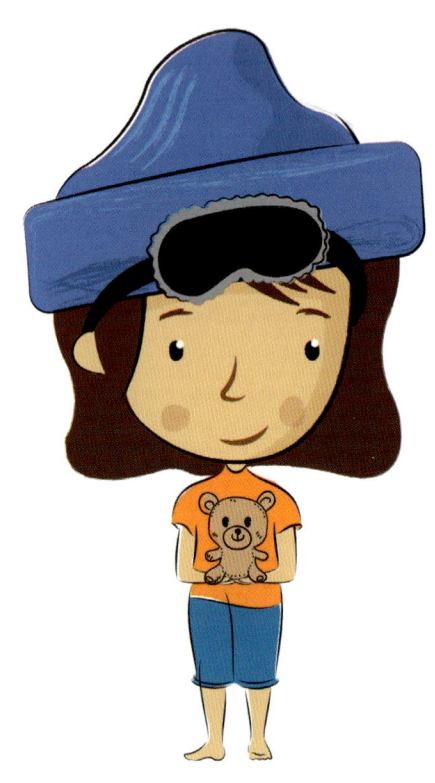

How else does yoga help?

It leads to deeper sleep.

It improves your mood.

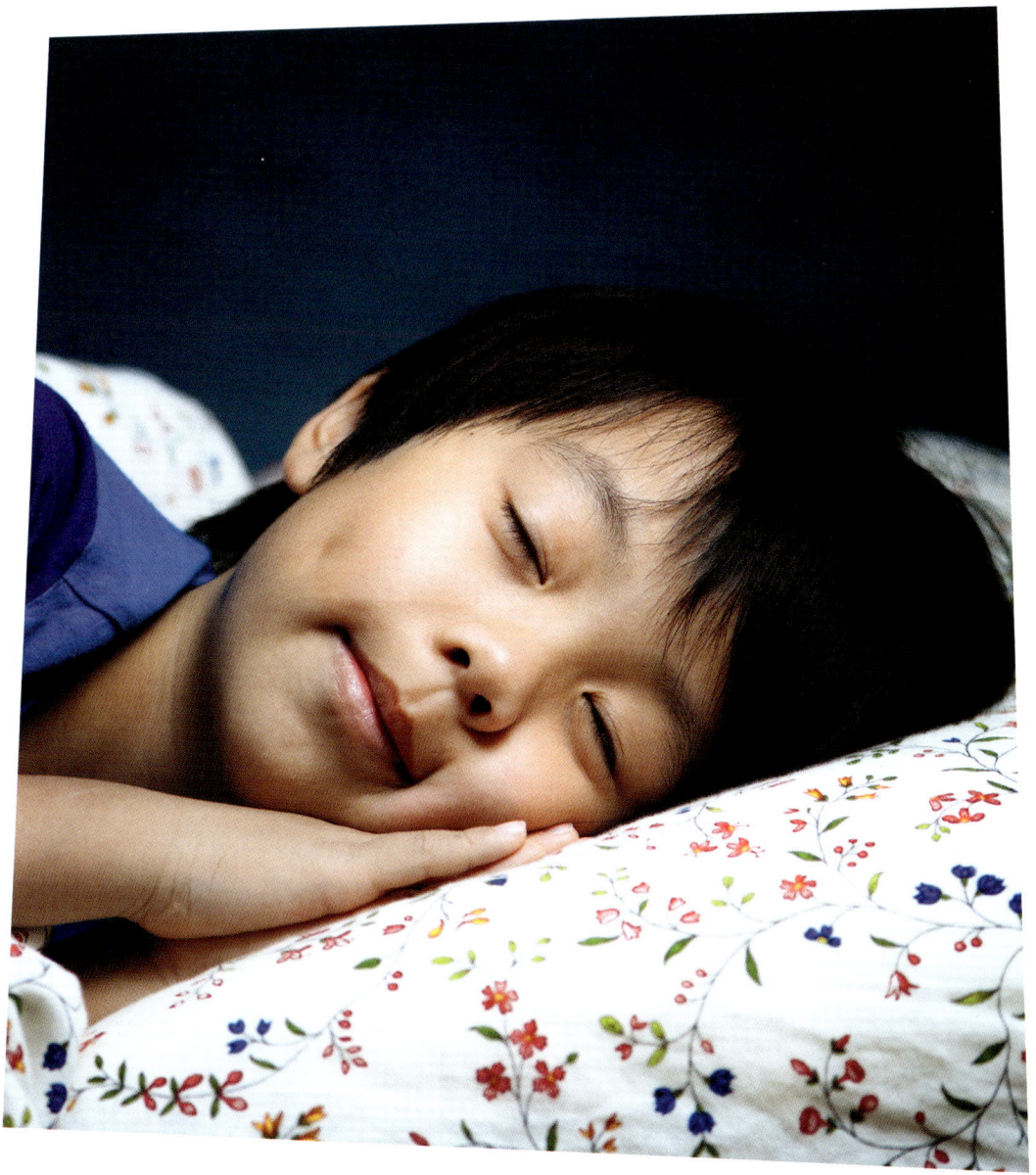

Yoga builds muscle.

It makes bones stronger.

Yoga even helps ease some pain.

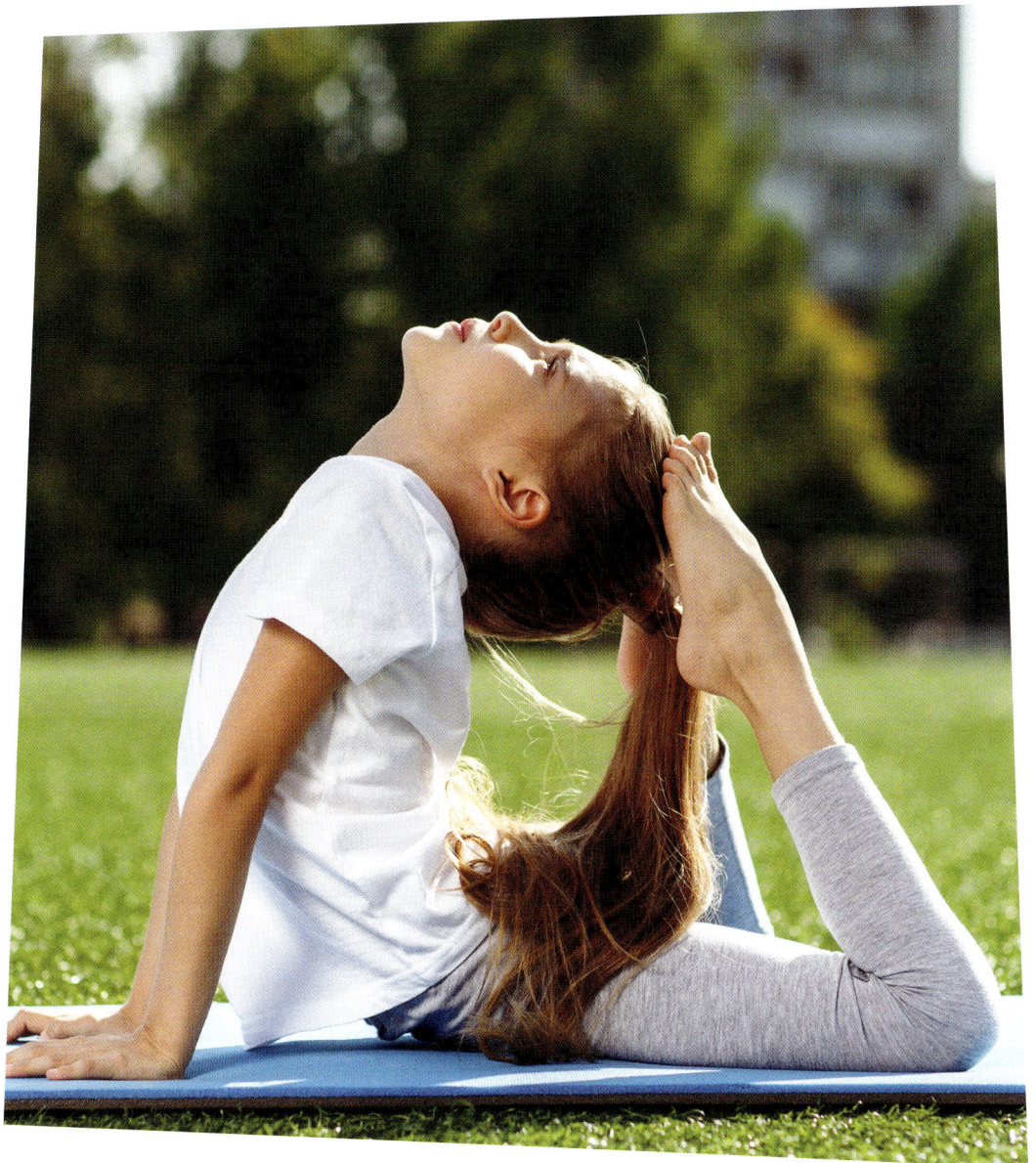

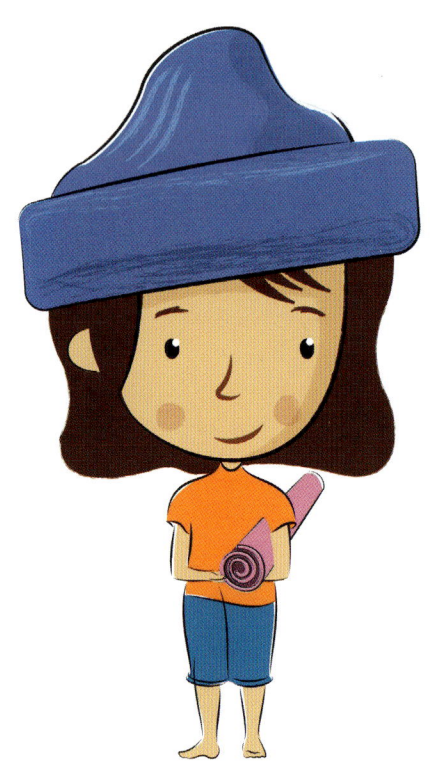

Find time for yoga during the day.

Even 15 minutes helps.

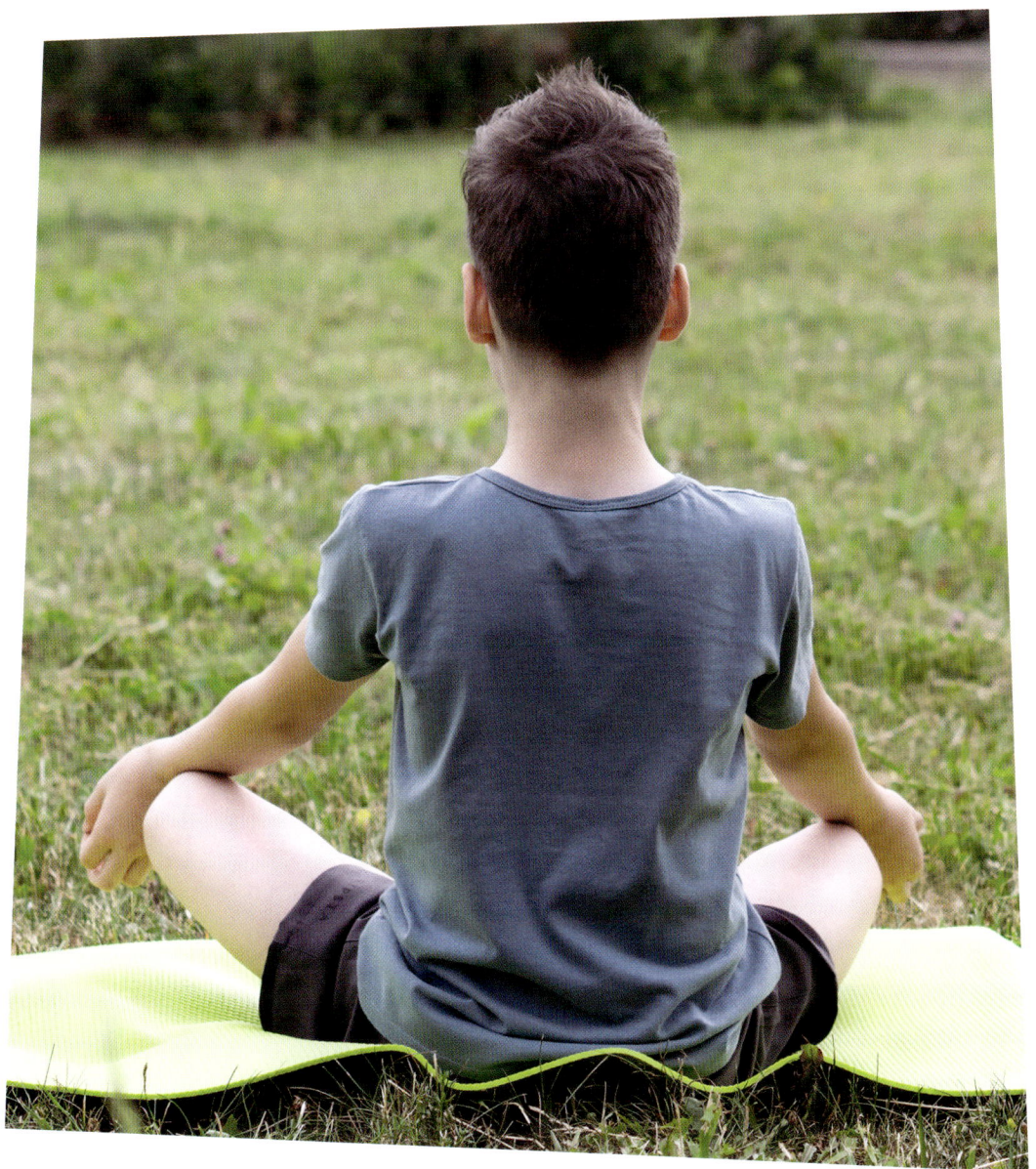

Life is busy.

You need to have focus.

But you want to feel good.

Yoga strikes a balance!

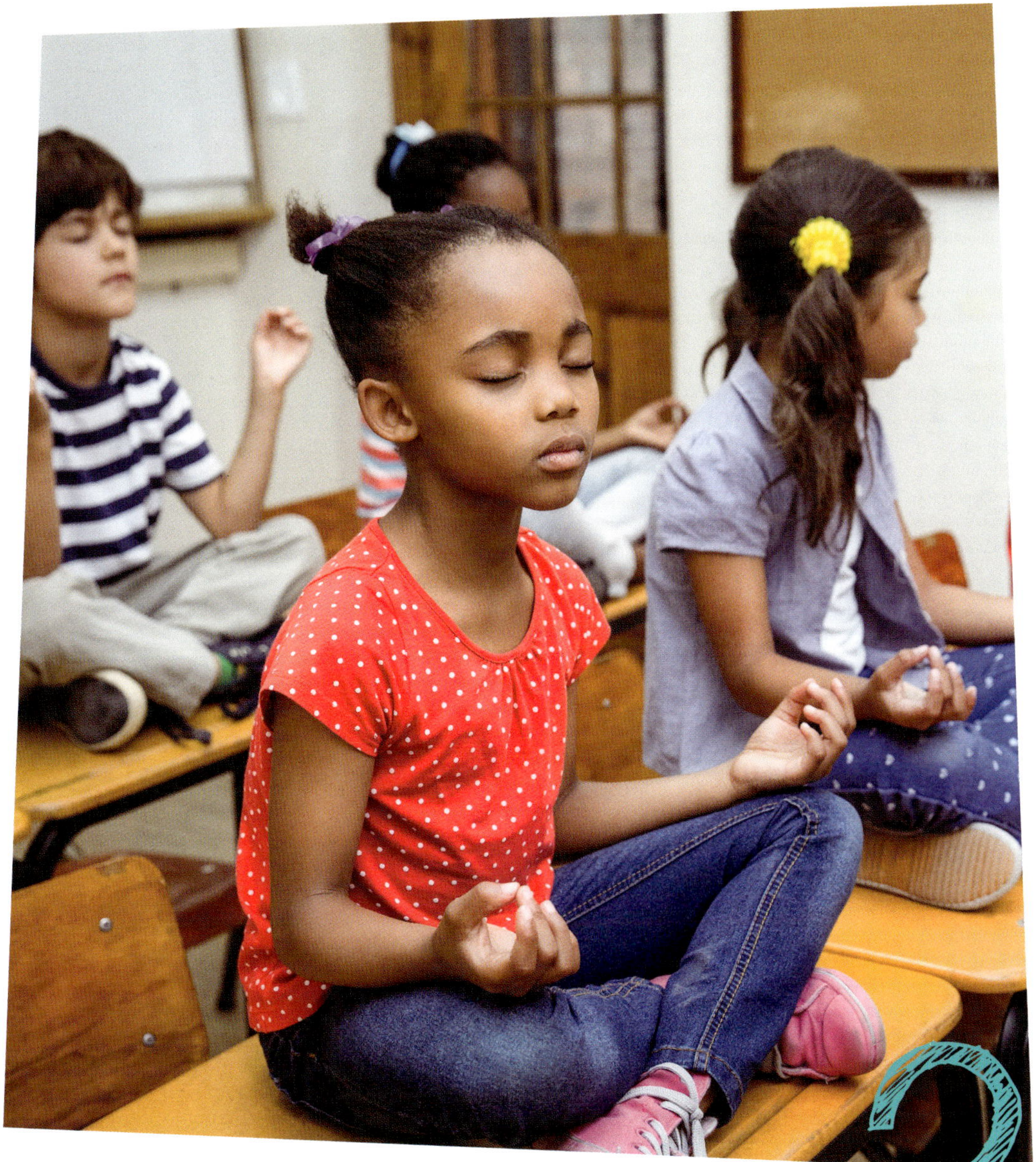

How can you be mindful today?

glossary & index

glossary

chant (CHANT) to sing or speak the same words over and over

focus (FOH-kuhs) to give your attention to

inner peace (IN-ur PEES) a quiet and calm state of mind

meditate (MED-ih-tate) to train your mind to relax and focus

mindful (MINDE-ful) aware of your body, mind, and feelings

pose (POHZ) the position in which someone sits or stands

random (RAN-duhm) without direction or purpose

relax (rih-LAKS) to take a rest from work or do something enjoyable

yoga (YOH-guh) poses, breathing, and sometimes meditation and chanting that provide balance and good health

index

balance, 8, 22

exercise, 8

focus, 14, 22

meditate, 14

mindful, 14, 23

pose, 4, 12, 13